A PHYSICIAN'S COUNSELS

TO HIS

PROFESSIONAL BRETHREN.

BY A PRACTISING PHYSICIAN.

PHILADELPHIA:
PRESBYTERIAN BOARD OF PUBLICATION,
NO. 821 CHESTNUT STREET.

STEREOTYPED BY
JESPER HARDING & SON,
INQUIRER BUILDING, SOUTH THIRD STREET, PHILADELPHIA.

PREFACE.

THIS little treatise has been prepared by its author, with the humble desire of drawing the attention of medical men to their religious privileges and responsibilities on the one hand, and the temptations which assail them on the other. No one can trace our profession, in the retrospect of past ages, without feeling its barrenness of a general, vital, moral power. As a body we have too often seen it incredulous and sceptical; and even in a time of enlightenment we find Sir Thomas Browne, in his "Religio Medici," writing as if it were almost necessary for a physician to apologize for having any orthodox views. Such a state of things has in part passed away, and the genial warmth of true science and revelation has melted and floated off many of the barriers which, like arctic icebergs, impeded moral progress. Still there is a want of applied, earnest, concentrated, religious influence, which we believe investigation, and a sense of our spiritual duty and accountability, will develope. In communicating with considerate and intelligent men, the chief point is to lead them to think for themselves, on the subject introduced for their consideration; and with the earnest hope that these few pages may accomplish this, I dedicate them

TO THE

FRATERNITY OF

MEDICINE.

May 1859.

CONTENTS.

CHAPTER I.

CHAPTER II.

A PHYSICIAN'S COUNSELS.

TO HIS

PROFESSIONAL BRETHREN.

CHAPTER I.

The importance of the medical profession—what its religious influence and tendencies—the study and practice full of materials for religious contemplation—religious truths enforced by it in its various departments—it addresses itself to our immortal natures—suggestive of serious thought—so far as it reaches, corroborative of reason and revelation—our need in it and as shown by it of relief and reliance above ourselves—the source and remedy.

THE practitioner of the healing art has, in all ages, attracted the attention of humanity. Man had not long emerged from his paradisiacal home, before disease, pain, and death assailed him, and suffering nature sought for relief and aid from medicines administered by those who professed to have learned their efficacy and curative powers. For a long period, like every infant science, medicine groped amid superstition and darkness; and with tradition and imperfect experience as its unsafe guides, became obscured by inaccurate experiments and assumed results. Imagination and credulity, in the absence of real knowledge, regarded the healing art with profound respect. Temples were erected to the curing gods, and panaceas and elixirs sought not only to overcome the sufferings of earth, but to set aside the stern decrees of death, by imparting the charms of a perennial and unfading life even on earth.

The healers of the sick were approached with veneration, and multitudes acknowledged their claims to extended influence. The disseminated light of learning, and the intelligent appreciation of the skilful Physician, secure to him a higher position and a more reasonable confidence. The human structure has been studied as a wondrous organism, in itself a cabinet of created wonders; while the sciences of nature, now viewed in their relation to, and bearing upon, our physical and moral welfare, afford regions of research of high attraction and noble extent. The physician, educated as he should be, assumes a high place and rank among the learned professions. Surrounded by such inducements to mental culture, and with the additional incentives afforded by the calls and necessities of the afflicted, a fair proportion of our educated men choose this as the occupation of their lives. The Christian, as he surveys the moral condition of the world, with no little solicitude inquires on which side, in the great conflict between right and wrong, religion and vice, truth and error, such a trained army is enlisted. Can the moralist, the philanthropist, and the Christian feel assured that this important profession is friendly to revealed religion, and that they who, by their daily business, declare the necessity for attention to the body, recognize the wants of the soul? Have they, who so often here behold the dire penalty of sin, provided themselves with the antidote to spiritual death? There is balm in Gilead, and a physician there; and while we administer to others for the cure of physical ills, shall we acquire no skill in ministering to a mind diseased? What are the special religious tendencies of medical education and practice? What its peculiar privileges, the special temptations to which it is exposed, and the special encouragements to associate it with a religious faith? Questions such as these must suggest themselves to the Christian physician, as deserving to be carefully considered by those who conscientiously desire to promote the moral advancement of their profession and their own spiritual welfare.

Will you not, my medical friend, bear with one of your own profession who, from the labours of active medical life, appropriates a little time to the consideration of these momentous questions? The very study of medicine opens up before the mind a field glowing with a harvest of suggestive religious contemplation. Man himself is the theme—creation's masterpiece, moulded from a heavenly original, who in his mere physical conformation, with which we have to deal, is a mechanical wonder. The phlegmatic Novalis, stirred into touching enthusiasm by the study, remarked, "There is but one temple in the universe, and that is the body of man. We touch heaven, when we lay hold on a human form." From this source Theology has drawn some of its most convincing proofs of a superior and designing intelligence; and the student, who, in the primal steps of his profession, has to do with its nice anatomical arrangements, cannot but recognize the proof and power of a divine origination. That heart with valves and countervalves, with reservoirs and aqueducts, in principle a perpetual motion; those lungs of a million little air cells, laboratories of God's chemistry; the eye with its lenses and its humours, its motions and its nerves, the great optic of the soul; the ear so nicely chiselled out, commencing with convoluted folds without, and transmitting the sound-waves through its labyrinth until it communicates with a world within; the muscles moving quickly responsive to the will, the bone and brain, globule and atom, taste and touch, matter and mind; oh! how, as hour after hour of research reveals to us facts and forms, adaptations and constructions, principles and skill, unseen by all around, do these speak to us of presiding goodness, wisdom, and love! While Bell can find in a human hand a fruitful subject for a Bridgewater treatise, to us the whole body is a museum of equal wonders.

If ever design proves a designer, law a lawmaker, skill an author, or the attributes of a being are to be inferred from the greatness of his works, then there is a forcible demonstration in the minutiæ of our daily study of a God who "made and fashioned us."

As we pass from the examination of the instrument to its functions, no less touching and impressive are the lessons taught. The entire physiology of life, assimilation, nutrition, reparation, decay,—all are as wonderful as the medium of transformation, and it requires no irrelevant effort, no turning aside from our pathway to behold omnipotent skill ruling over all; and although we study the laws of growth, and trace matter to its formative corpuscles and cell-atoms, yet, with all our investigations we find no creating, vitalizing power.

The physician, in the ardent study of his profession, with its kindred sciences, may imagine that he is on the verge of creative agency as he gets down to primitive cellules and finds their chemical construction; but here he must stop to acknowledge that the ability to make that atom, and breathe the breath of life within it is beyond all human power. Man the great investigator, and God the great Creator, are the twin mottoes stamped in impress deep upon the study of our art. But the moral grandeur of our pursuit is not hemmed in even by the wide range of self. The natural world, in connection with the human body, opens its rocks and its floras, its structure and its laws, to our view; and nicety of adaptation, and wisdom of design invite our notice and admiration at every turn.

As the natural eye looks abroad upon the

2

works of Deity, it is not difficult for the serious and contemplative to have the moral affections heightened and developed by the touching views of created objects that extend around us; but just as the microscopist sees in a raindrop beauties unknown, and unadmired by the unaided sight, so we find matter more perfect in her ultimate divisions than in the outlines of huge form, and thus are bound by more exquisite and golden chains to the unseen and immortal.

When we pass to the practice of the profession, and mingle this with our daily research, we find ourselves observers and reasoners upon the great facts of human existence. Ours is not the knowledge of the cloister, the studio, or the secluded book-room; but we are at once thrust out in contact with the great heart of real life, living witnesses of the illustrated commentary which observation affords upon the facts of revealed religion.

We behold this bodily machine in construction accurate, unique, reparative, perfect, yet suffering, exhausting, dying, and we feel that some strange discord has marred the symmetry of this wondrous instrument; that some after shock jarred the mechanism constructed for perpetual endurance. So marked is this, that some anatomists, exulting in the harmony, have zealously asserted that there is no reason why man should not live, and live on coeval with time, if he would but accurately obey the fundamental laws of life. But the fact of a temporary existence here outstrips and contradicts the argument; and as we see the strong man and the valiant bending before disease, or succumbing to the stern monitor; and as in ungoverned appetites or passions, or in the inherited diseases of former generations, we trace the causes of decay, we join our testimony corroborative of holy writ, that man, though perfect in his creation, has fallen from his high estate, and, with Milton, sorrowfully mourn that sin "brought death into the world and all our woe."

The sick and suffering we conjure to seek for aid from sources extrinsic to themselves, and often, in our own experience, realize the total inefficiency of human power even in physical ailments. Shall we not then learn to look to some higher source for deliverance from that inward malady, which, unchecked by mere human agency, corrodes and permeates the soul?

In the daily walks of our profession, how many serious and truthful lessons force themselves upon our attention! Here is the palace of the rich, surrounded by all the luxuries and charms that earthly treasures can impart; but in that almost regal home lies a human sufferer, whom wealth and elegance fail to soothe. Disease, pain, and death, unbidden stalk amid the magnificence of earth, and teach the physician more potently than others, because the contrast is more frequently thrust upon his notice, that we must look for true and lasting happiness above and beyond the world around us, to a spring perennial on high, unaffected by the turbidness of earth. As, perchance, you have passed from such a scene to some lonely cottage, or falling hovel, where everything betokens want and destitution, and looked on some other sufferer, submissive, uncomplaining, happy, with eye beaming with eternal hope, and heart resting on the "Friend that sticketh closer than a brother;" have you never felt that there is a power in that religion which reverses the fortunes of men, and irradiates the darkened chamber of sickness with the light and consolation of a spiritual hope? In the diverse allotments too of men, we cannot but read the proofs of a future retributive justice. As we survey the home field of life, we recognize that the condition of different members of the human race is out of all proportion to their characters and conduct, and that the penalty of sin, though visited on all, bears not here exact proportion to the amount of demerit, while we see a finger pointing beyond to a judgment according to desert. Our very calling has in it a divine philosophy teaching, by experience and by example, as well as by the facts of revelation, the power and necessity of faith. No one, we may certainly say, has the same opportunity to learn from nature, and from practical life the great facts of human existence so readily as the physician. He has to do with the inner current of society, and that too not in its smooth and placid hours, but when rippled and agitated by anxiety and fear. Where others look upon the outside circle of enchantment, it is his to stand bending over the whirlpool into which ere long the hopes of present life are engulfed; and where the passing world sees only a surface of happiness to be envied, or of misery to be deplored, the physician has an inner view which modifies the picture. In the buoyancy of health, man seems strong, independent, magnanimous, and is apt to feel himself a Hercules in self-reliant power, and to forget his trust on superhuman aid; but on us the prostrate form, the helpless call, the feeble voice most powerfully impress the daily sermon that we are weak, dependent creatures, and can do but little to save even ourselves from present malady. The communings of our business are often with life's shadows, and as the absence of the full ray on a part of the plate of the daguerreotype makes the perfect picture; so, to our observation the mingling of lights and shades makes up the faithful portraiture of life.

And then there is *death*, to others an unfamiliar object in its details, but to us a frequent messenger summoning us to its presence-chamber, and calling on us to preside over the last muffled heart-beat of its triumph. As you are called upon to behold the strong man laid low, and touch the final pulse of one but a little while before ruddy with healthful life; or as at dead of night you leave the home where just now the closing breath has told you that your effort is at an end; and the silent street or lonely country road echoes to your passage; do not serious thoughts obtrude themselves upon your mind? What is life? May not the next call I receive be that of death, a messenger to me? Am I prepared to pass through such a scene, myself being the subject? Have I the Rock of ages for my refuge? or must I then endure the dark forebodings with which I have known others look down into the tomb. Is it wise to spend our days in seeking honours and treasures here, forgetful of these trying hours, which are forerunners of an everlasting future? The physician, who dares to think, cannot, it would seem, fail to ponder the questions of solemn and eternal import which his occupation suggests; and to none does a more frequent or more touching voice cry out, "Prepare to meet thy God."

Procrastination too is out of all keeping with the acquired habits of our lives. In medical experience we appreciate the often critical danger of delay. A quick perception of the necessities of the case, decision in judgment, and promptness in execution, constitute no unimportant attributes of the successful practitioner. Appreciating the value of the present *now* in reference to the body, shall we forget its still more pressing importance in its relation to the soul? Most men, if they knew the precise day and hour in which they would be summoned to exchange the scenes of time for the unalterable destiny of eternity, would set apart a certain period for preparation for this untried future; but, since we know it not, and oft repeated cases have proved to us that it may be very near at hand; how much more reasonable that the time for preparation be the present! None learn so forcibly as we, what an unfavourable and unseasonable opportunity sickness affords for calm and deliberate thought upon the interests of our souls. How often, as we review the practice of the past, do these death-bed scenes file in array before us; and what instruction do they impart, as to the utter folly of hoping to make ready for eternity in the anxious and disturbed season which precedes departure!

The man of wealth, with will and testament unmade, you feel it to be a duty to apprize of his condition, and counsel him to make arrangements for the crisis. Anxious, perturbed, and perhaps racked with pain, it is difficult to fix his attention even on these earthly things; prostration and returning pangs interrupt the communication of his views, and with difficulty the last desires are expressed. But how much more hopeless to commence preparation for the dying hour and the retributions of the future, when nature is fast sinking into decay! Not to procure a life boat until the flood is overwhelming us, not to effect an insurance until the frame work is in flames, and the whirlwind fanning it! Oh! the utter folly of postponing the great business of life to its suffering terminus. No scene meets us in life more distressing than a diseased body writhing under the additional agonies of a terror-stricken soul; the future darker than death, or lurid with the flames of a guilty and exasperated conscience. As I heard a friend speak of eternity to such a one, and saw him turn his face to the wall to die, while his pallid lips cried out, "Don't mention it; don't mention it;" those eyes ghastly with intensity, and that countenance haggard with foreboding, left on my mind an impression which during life cannot be effaced. Death-bed repentances, when nature is "frightened into propriety," or when the pressure of existing trouble makes us think, give but a quivering, hesitating hope; and of all mankind who postpone immortal interests to the last, the physician is the most inexcusable. His life-work, made forcible by impressive examples, is his accusing monitor. Let the stammering accent of each final whisper, from patients groping in the valley of death, admonish us, "Be ye also ready, for in such an hour as ye think not the Son of man cometh."

But not only at the closing point of life, and in common with all mankind, does the physician need the consolations of religion, but in the very practice and trials of his profession he may well desire its solace. There are periods in the experience of the most skilled when the feeling of personal responsibility weighs down the spirits; when we hesitate in guiding the life-canoe amid the rapids which threaten it; when the patient clings to us as his main support, and we feel the need of some higher power to impart efficacy to our efforts. Not many years ago I met in the crowded street a physician who had lost two children of a family, by croup, in as many days, and now the third was hopelessly struggling for life.

As he mentioned to me the circumstances, and exhibited the sympathy of his own afflicted heart, "Ah!" said he, "I am not in the habit of praying, but the parents asked me to pray for them, and if ever a person prayed in earnest, I did." There are occasions when we need consolation as well as the bereaved, when we cannot stay the hand of the destroyer, or when perchance ill deserved censure is the reward of our best efforts, or when death startles us by its suddenness, and the greatest of all consolations is to have an omniscient, almighty, and willing Friend on whom we can rely and to whom we can repair.

There are many considerations, addressing themselves to the reason and conscience, or suggested by the word of God and such works as those of Baxter, Doddridge, Venn, and Alleine, which would seem sufficient to draw all men to Christ, and of which, in common with all others, we should avail ourselves, but our object is to direct attention particularly to the considerations which are daily suggested by our professional pursuits.

If the poet, from a contemplation of the phenomena of nature, could justly and pointedly pronounce "the undevout astronomer mad;" with equal point and truth it might be affirmed of the undevout physician.

Anatomy, Physiology, Physics, rationally studied, point with unerring finger to a great first Cause, who claims our homage and the expression of our gratitude and love. Each day's experience and observation declare to us that human nature labours under a malady which no medicine can cure, and for the relief of which the resort must be to a higher than mortal power. To Christ, the great Physician, we may come, with the assurance that he will be our healer. The disease is desperate but easily recognized, the remedy is accessible, and the principles and habits of our profession would suggest the immediate application of the remedy.

Truth and not fancy thus portrays our case:

"Deep are the wounds which sin has made,
 Where shall the sinner find a cure?

In vain, alas! is nature's aid,
  The work exceeds all nature's power.

Sin, like a raging fever, reigns
  With fatal strength in every part,
The dire contagion fills the veins,
  And spreads its poison to the heart.

And can no sovereign balm be found?
  And is no kind physician nigh,
To ease the pain and heal the wound,
  Ere life and hope for ever fly?

There is a great Physician near,
  Look up, O fainting soul, and live;
See, in his heavenly smiles appear
  Such aid as nature cannot give.

See, in the Saviour's dying blood,
  Life, health, and bliss abundant flow;
'Tis only this pure sacred flood
  Can ease thy pain and heal thy wo."

CHAPTER II.

Hindrances to a religious life, and temptations peculiar to our profession—science in its first conceptions often tends to scepticism—effect of French morals and doctrine—materialism—erroneous conclusions as to truth from false arguments—the hardening influence of familiarity with trying scenes—errors of practice—secularization of the Sabbath—irregularity of life—licentiousness of conduct or conversation—other temptations in common with all.

In the previous chapter, we have glanced at the peculiar illustration and enforcement which religion receives from our profession, in addition to the numerous and general inducements which address themselves to all who would participate in its benefits. Men, however, are disposed to shelter themselves under the hindrances which may be supposed to arise from their peculiar vocations; and these, whether feigned or real, are worthy of distinct consideration.

At the very outset of the inquiry, we are met with the serious allegations that the tendency of the study of medicine is unfriendly to personal piety. It has been affirmed, that there is more scepticism and loose morality in our profession than among any other single class of literary or professional men; and the physician cannot but feel disposed, either upon evidence to deny the charge, or else upon facts and principles to exhibit the cause of this anomaly. That such has been, to a limited extent, the fact, must be admitted; but that such is not at present the case, and that where existing it has been owing to other than medical causes, or to illogical deductions from just premises, will we think be evident to all who look for the real source of the difficulty. To any one who, without irreligious prejudices, has studied the symmetry and harmony of our corporeal natures, and the laws which govern its relationship to the outer world, and who has sought to learn and profit by the lessons of his practical experience, the presumption is at once that the reason for special moral delinquencies in our art, if such exist, must be sought outside the sphere of pure medical truth.

Two facts are to be taken into consideration in reviewing the medico-religious character of the past, with its waning influence on the present.

The spirit of scientific inquiry, the disposition to reason out everything, and to subject all things to this test, always has a tendency towards scepticism, and it is only when the ultimatum of the truth has been attained, and the whole field of argument can be carefully surveyed by well-trained, well-balanced logical minds, that these imagined contradictions are found to be "oppositions of science falsely so called." More than once have even good and great men trembled at their own conclusions, apparently irreconcilable with revealed truth; but on further investigation light has shone upon their pathway and proved their reasoning fallacious. Science, proudly and rightfully exultant in its triumphs, is sometimes too prone to bring religion to its test, rather than consider itself as subject to be tried by its loftier superior. We have a right to ask and expect that these be found in beautiful and unconflicting correspondence, so far as they deal with subjects within their mutual grasp; but when the human mind in the glow and flush of high reason, forgets its stopping point, and with the analogies and scales of time, attempts to try and weigh the materials of faith and eternity, it chases a horizon which will illimitably recede.

In a study like that of medicine, pursued as it too often is by those whose minds, by previous discipline, have not been thoroughly prepared for logical analysis, there is constant danger of falling into this very error. Of all the practical sciences it is the most varied, inquisitive, suggestive, and explorative; and enlisting almost every natural science as an accessary in its eager pathway sometimes falls upon erroneous conclusions. Discovery after discovery, as to the laws of existence, have followed each other so rapidly as scarcely to allow opportunity for close analysis; and what on superficial view appears to be the natural sequence of cause and effect, overthrowing established belief, under severer scrutiny proves itself mere analogical assumption.

Another incidental occasion of medical scepticism cannot be overlooked. The atmosphere in which medical education formerly attained its highest perfection, was unfriendly to simplicity of religious faith. France has long been the centre of attraction to the student of medicine, and Parisian morals and scepticism could not but exert their evil power over the unprotected student. The popular philosophy of Voltaire and Rousseau, gilded with the sophistry and sustained by the literary fame of its authors, lured the youthful physician within its meshes, and many students returned to the homes of their boyhood, tainted and corrupted from this source, and not, as alleged, by their strictly medical education. The ingenuous and inexperienced student, removed from home influences, was peculiarly exposed to their malign associations, and if infected it was due to the weakness of human nature, and not to any sinister influence of his medical pursuits.

The peculiar form of scepticism into which the medical student is most liable to be betrayed, is known under the designation of materialism; a dogma so fascinating that many have been deluded by it, who, on calm reflection, would be startled by the consequences to which it inevitably leads. While, in effect, it excludes God from the universe, it regards with seeming reverence the works of nature, so called, which derive all their significancy from the fact that they are the visible representatives of God's creating power and wisdom. The materialist sees in matter a self-propagating, self-governing, and indeed a self-originating power. It refers all the phenomena of existence to what are called the laws of nature, as in themselves sufficient for their production; and investing these material laws with an intrinsic potency, it finds no place for spiritual existence. The soul of man is a material soul, subject to all the vicissitudes of the material body. In ascertaining the laws of growth and transformation, and witnessing the wonderful reparative powers of nature, he is illogically led to what are called ultimate axioms, and to the ascription of creative energy to material atoms. Deliberate reason is often made to succumb to the enthusiasm of the student who pries into the mysteries of the human organism; and while contemplating the perfect structure, the divine Constructor is ignored as an object of faith. It seems to be forgotten that reasoning from the objects of sight may mislead, and that testimony and consciousness may be true sources of knowledge as well as experiment and observation.

The materialistic theory is surrounded by difficulties. If the laws impressed on matter are to be substituted in the place of God, the question will still recur, How did those laws originate, and how is their continuance perpetuated? Did they come by chance, and are they continued by chance? If there be anything which may be called chance, it can possess no such regularity and seeming intelligence; but if chance be "direction which we cannot see," then we come back to the idea of a supreme intelligence which has made and controls all things. We may talk of material power, law, and order, the sequence of cause and effect, but they have no meaning unless we place back of them an intelligent first cause. The materialism which ignores God as the great presiding spirit, leads to the denial of our own spiritual existence, in defiance of our own consciousness, and the many facts which can alone be accounted for on the admission of spiritual existence. In adopting the materialistic view we must not only dethrone God from his universe; debase our own nature by denying its higher principles and bring it down to the level of the brute; repudiate a divine revelation, bearing such credentials of its heavenly origin, so animating to our hopes, and so soothing to our sorrows; but we must contradict our own practice. Where else do we recognize matter without a maker? Where, in art, is our admiration of a structure so absorbing as to lose sight of its author and designer? How does it happen that the greater the perfection of execution, the more zealously we seek and admire the designing intelligence? Shall we applaud the sculptor of some nicely chiselled form, and never ask for Him who made the speaking, thinking, acting, moving model? We have machines in art, which, not only transform the article committed to them in a single particular, and pass it from one state of change to another, but which even provide for the contingencies of accident; yet in reviewing the wonderful processes, we do not lose sight of the inventor, or attribute to the thing made inherent wisdom or design.

In the human frame, we see wonderful proofs of skill, and of reparative power, of application and subservience to well-established laws; we admire changes the most unique, and modifications of matter the most wonderful; but yet have you ever known an atom from nothing create itself? We dissect and philosophize man down to what we term his ultimate constituents, and strive to determine his chemical affinities, and the exact proportions of minerals and gases that form him; but how near have any of us come to manufacturing a single drop of the life blood that circulates through his veins? We must not, in the use of such terms as elementary, primitive, primary, ultimate, and the like, deceive ourselves into the idea that in matter we have arrived at the fundamentals of all construction. These are but relative and conventional terms by which we measure the limit of our knowledge. The wonderful combinations and transformations of material in the human frame, with all the functions elaborated thereby, are just as far from origination, creation, divinity, as the kaleidoscope, with its changing forms and varied colours, is from making the glass and the light-rays on which these depend. The state of the human system, as we find it, gives but little encouragement to the notion of what materialists call the natural, originating, progressive powers of matter. To say the least, it has done nothing in this line for man in our day. The heart beats no more synchronously, the blood circulates no more evenly than when Harvey first beheld it coursing through the veins; the lungs perform their part no better because we understand the physiology of respiration, and the brain is no more active since we have come to the fibriles of the nerves. We have seen a blood corpuscle break down, resolve itself into its constituents, and new ones forming from the fresh material supplied, but have never yet been able to recognize thought as a specific function, or to measure the diameter of the soul-atoms of which it is constructed; and if matter is everything, it is strange that we have never seen the *will* with the microscope, caught an *idea* in the process of physical elimination, or touched a *thought* in its material circulation.

Struck by the want of evidence which materialism in its full fledged form exhibits, and by the negations it requires, few medical men of the present day find reason from their study to adopt its difficult philosophy; but some still find refuge in its more modified and accommodating form, which, while less objectionable and more plausible, is yet rigid and forbidding.

These admit an author to creation, a great original, incomprehensible I AM, but yet deny to him any concern in the actual affairs of the universe. Placing him back at the final outposts of a past infinity, they regard him as starting all things in their motions, and instituting perfect laws to govern them, and then retiring from control, and leaving all to move in their ordained and everlasting courses. This, to say the least, is all assumption. We cannot admit a being with power to create and originate, without also granting him the power of an omnipresent view of, and control over, every thing transpiring among created objects. Infinity once admitted, we cannot limit it. It is probable that he who made all things would exercise an oversight; and even should we find for every organ and function, a well defined law according to which its results were attained, it would only show a non-interference, not his absence. What reason does not disprove, faith, consciousness, and revelation are fully competent to establish; and abundant are the evidences from these of God's active government, and his particular providence exercised over the affairs of men. He has chosen to make law and order the rule in the kingdoms of nature, but now and then he may choose to exceed, modify, or suspend them. Even death may occur as the result of what we call natural causes, and yet be a providential visitation. Twelve men in full health are exposed together, in a boat, to precisely similar influences, and of these, eight receive a severe cold, while four escape. Of the eight, one has peritonitis, another rheumatism, another pneumonia, another pleurisy, and two of the most healthy die. Now, although we may be able to discover each fatal pathological condition, and to account scientifically for their deaths, as a result of physical laws; yet, how totally unable are we to tell why the others did not meet the same fate! Then again, men die when the most skilled are totally unable to assign a cause, even after the most rigid autopsy, and others escape when they cannot conceive how; and thus, although in the death of persons the laws of nature are fulfilled, yet, while the modes, so to speak, are incidentally legal, the result is nevertheless designedly providential. With many it is professional always to assign a cause, and though it may be satisfactory to friends, we must not by the habit mislead ourselves. Behind each reason given there is something hidden, which when considered will lead us to the recognition of the present controlling power of God. Investigate and admire the symmetry of the laws which concern ourselves as we may, they are not adequate to the explanation of every psychological or moral fact. Medical reasoning and minute investigation are commendable, when they cling to what they see and know; and matter itself, in its changing forms and combinations, is worthy of our highest admiration; but we have never learned to make of it a soul, or endow it with celestial attributes. We cannot, we ought not, to bid adieu to the noble hopes, the lofty aspirations, the long settled beliefs, the powerful convictions, the revealed truths of our holy religion, not disproved by any course of logical reasoning, and receive in their stead an imaginary idea of a matter-manufactured system.

Another temptation to which the physician is exposed is that of drawing erroneous conclusions as to revealed truth from the imperfect proofs sometimes adduced in its support. Theological writers, and ministers more frequently in sermons, sometimes employ illogical arguments to establish religious doctrines which stand in no need of such support; and the hearer, detecting the fallacy of the reasoning, is apt therefrom to doubt the correctness of the premises. Inferences are drawn from the frame work and the phenomena with which the medical man has to deal, and he therefore is more acute to detect the fallacy, and to draw his own unfavourable inferences. How frequently are pathetic accounts given of peaceful deaths, where the physician knows that that kind of termination was, and always is, characteristic of that form of disease; and of disturbed deaths where these again are incident to the malady, and to which the best men are liable. Supposed death-bed repentances have to him in cases of recovery so often proved spurious, and analogies from the material to the immaterial so often strike him correctly as erroneous, that it requires a constant guard lest, while others are enlarging upon these, his feelings be biased in a path prejudicial to the exercise of a saving faith. The antidote is at once simple, reasonable, efficacious, and complete. Never doubt a fact of revelation because you can answer a human argument in respect to it. Go back to that book, and that source where no sophistry can be detected, and with reason under proper control, not seeking to grasp too much, and with faith and feeling pliable to the power of truth, drink fresh and at first-hand from the gushing well-spring of divine knowledge. Instead of seeking to answer the word of man, and becoming sceptical by the success, it is safer and better to go directly to the word of God, and thus be refreshed and established from the pure fountain-head. It is a historical fact in the records of infidelity that few constant readers of the Bible, seeking after the truth, have ever swerved in their religious belief, while multitudes, who have been led astray by their own reasonings, or by the honest fallacies of imperfect expounders, have found the true way when they have studied for themselves the text-book without note or commentary. While too, in matters of observation, our own experience may neutralize the inferences from analogy, and from modes of death as described by others, yet where we do see religion triumphing with calm and holy resignation, where nature is strongest in its opposite tendencies—in such instances the moral lesson addresses itself to us more potently because of our knowledge, and furnishes an argument whose redoubled power we can well appreciate. Medical facts and information may not always confirm the explanations or illustrations of men; but so far as they reach will corroborate the testimony of natural and revealed religion as to the condition, the wants, and the destiny of the human race.

A third error of inference and belief to which medical men are exposed, is that derived from their peculiar relation to mankind in sickness and death, and from their constant familiarity with critical and solemn scenes. The physician meets the sick with a business air, in a business capacity, dealing with pain, disease, and death professionally; and thus events which alarm and distress some, and excite others, as well they may, to serious contemplation, become quite familiar to him in his formal official capacity. This irresistible power of habit exercises an influence over our thoughts which we cannot directly set aside. Even the Christian minister is exposed to it, and is in danger of lacking soul-piety and earnestness from his very familiarity with the language and routine of religious expression; or, as Dr. Holmes rather quaintly and strongly expresses it, is in danger of lapsing into heathenism from his preaching, and from the want of fresh religious instruction.

The philanthropist visiting prison houses, the poor-master in formal care for the pauper, the tract distributor for the destitute, will inevitably become hardened in their work, unless they balance the tendency by cultivating in turn the habit of sympathy and relief. The physician, having constantly to deal with human nature in its least attractive forms, and with its most solemn conditions, as one in authority, must and will be imperceptibly, yet surely, seared to proper feeling and impression, unless he too seeks the natural and only preservative, which is to cultivate a moral sense and an emotional sympathy, and thus neutralize one habit by another equally powerful. In reality, if we but think, we will feel that the blighting of human hopes is none the less real because we see it; pain and disease no less serious because our companions; and death to us personally no less certain, and if unprepared for no less absolutely terrible because we daily behold it; and reason therefore teaches us to improve these events to our own spiritual preparation, and to use them as we have before considered them to be, additional warnings rather than the occasion of hardening and steeling the soul. The power of one's occupation over his habits of thought, the necessity of recognizing it, and the means of overcoming it, are so forcibly discussed by Bishop Butler, author of the "Analogy," as to be well worthy of the notice of any one who does not realize the strength of his temptation.

If there are any other errors of religious belief which harass the mind of the physician, our own Dr. Nelson has most ably met them, in his "Cause and Cure of Infidelity;" and there are many other books in our English tongue, which, to educated men are easily accessible, and abundantly conclusive on these points. Without, therefore, seeking to compass the various general forms of scepticism, which attach with no special or peculiar power to our science and art, we pass from the beliefs to the demoralizing practices which may be engendered by our profession, unless we are on the watch to resist and overcome temptation.

The first we notice is a secularization of the Sabbath. Around this holy day centre the hopes, not only of religion, but also of morality; and even civil government needs the aid of its hallowed and protecting influence. Once the world witnessed the experiment of lessening its frequency, until, amid increasing tumult and wild uproar, a nation caring not for its sacred associations sought its restoration even as a police measure. Reared in a land where its obligations are admitted, we can scarcely appreciate the intimate connection its proper observance bears to our social and national well-being, and what a relation it holds to our own personal and individual stability of character. No one, even from apparent necessity, can habitually break over its restraints without lowering his standard of religious sensibility. No temptation assails even the more correct class of medical men more plausibly than this. Our business even comes under the exception of works of necessity and mercy, and there is no cessation of our daily avocation. The wants of the sick seem to make to us every day alike ; and the routine of our life has no seventh period as a resting point. Justified in public view by the calls of our profession, we walk, and drive, and visit, and carry on our occupation, feeling that what we do will not be judged as would the deeds of other men. I know, I speak the experience of many a physician when I express the longing we feel for this as a day of physical and mental rest, and of many a moral and Christian physician who laments the seeming necessity for labour, and the tendency it has to divert and interrupt the mind in the contemplation of things sacred and divine. Our standard of moral excellence must and will be lowered, unless we recognize the power of this evil to which we are exposed, and fortify ourselves against it. In common with others, we need the spiritual refreshment it affords, and the season it provides for meditation, reflection, Christian instruction, and public and private worship, and unless on the alert to improve what time we have, we shall suffer in our happiness here, and our everlasting welfare hereafter.

I am convinced that many of us, satisfied from habit of the necessity of attending to our business, do not redeem the time of the Sabbath as we might. Any one who has not tried the experiment will be surprised to find how much of it, by a little management, may be secured from mere professional labour. An extra diligence on Saturday afternoon and Monday morning, attendance to chronic cases on week days, a rising earlier upon the Sabbath instead of later than on other days, a more careful economizing of the hours will allow us much more of its rest and benefits than we suppose. Habit or carelessness often leads to a neglect in which we are not justified by an analysis of the amount of labour performed. I knew well a conscientious physician, who seldom attended church, as he really thought because his business would not permit of it, but his successor attending to a practice fully as great was as rarely absent. During the cholera season in New York city my attention was attracted, on the Sabbath, to a gentleman who, though often a little late, was rarely absent from his place in the sanctuary; and on inquiry I found him to be a medical man who was said by those of his own profession, familiar with him, to visit as many patients per day as any physician in the city. The time is past when it is politic to attempt to advertize our immense popularity and practice by staying away from the means of grace. Exceptions must and will occur, but the doctor who, as a rule, is not able to attend once on the Sabbath upon public worship, either does not properly economize his time, is not anxious enough to attend, or his business and moral welfare require that he should seek a partner.

But the physician upon the Sabbath has Christian duties and privileges outside of the great congregation. It is possible to remember the Sabbath day to keep it holy, even in the midst of our professional avocations, nay more, it is a duty. Heavenly contemplation should be our companion; and our sedateness of conduct on that day, while not austere, should impress those on whom we call that we know it to be the Sabbath. Our serious demeanour and avoidance of secular conversation will impart an influence which will affect those about us as does the gentle dew the needy plant. The fourth commandment is exceedingly broad, and its requirements are more imperative on us than we are apt to realize; and many excuses, I fear, which now our profession induces to make, will not stand the test of final scrutiny. If necessity compels us to go about, let us go about doing good, ministering to the soul as well as to the body where circumstances will admit, with our thoughts on heaven as well as upon the earth, sanctifying the teachings of sorrow, sickness, and death. We cannot afford better than others to lose the blessings of thought, and rest, and spiritual growth to which this day is favourable; and by how much they are imperiled by the secular character of our duties, by so much should we watch to overcome the tendency, and divert it into the channel of positive good. Let the Sabbath be to us holy, a delight, honourable, and besides securing greater comfort to ourselves, the example will tell for good upon those in whom neglect seems less excusable.

Next there is a natural disposition to irregularity in the duties and habits of life, which is apt to be fostered by the character of our profession, and in respect to which we need to be on our guard. The disorderly, unsystematic person will be inefficient in his moral duties as well as in business employments, and order is as important to spiritual as it is to physical, mental, or pecuniary prosperity. It cannot be denied that perfect system and symmetry are very difficult, and sometimes impossible to be secured in the practice of the physician. Unseasonable calls and unexpected detentions will sometimes overturn his best arranged plans. This too often furnishes an excuse even to the conscientious for the neglect of some of the every day duties of life. Here again methodical effort will often overcome apparent obstacles. It was said of Boerhaave that, notwithstanding his immense daily labour, he almost always found time for his hour of private worship, saying that "for the interests of his patients as well as himself he could not afford to intermit so important an exercise." In our family and more public weekly religious observances, we need a constant supervision lest our business be made an apology for neglect, when really, if some high enjoyment were in question, we would so arrange our duties as to avail ourselves of it. Where there is a will, even in our profession, there is more likely to be a way; and with a desire to do and to get good we will be oftener found in our appropriate places than many who have less to detain them. No one has a better opportunity than the consistent practitioner, to leave the impress of his character upon the community in which he dwells, and he should be careful that this stamp shall be one which he will not be ashamed to recognize when the great seal shall be set upon his works.

Licentiousness, either of conduct or conversation, is a temptation to which the unguarded physician may be exposed; but when we take a view of his position in society, of the sacred trusts committed to his keeping, and the high obligations imposed upon him, we cannot but recognize the marked incongruity between his profession and such principles or actions, and look with mingled pity and disgust upon those who have not the moral courage and self-respect to maintain, in the practice of their art, purity of language and of life. Though we may have to deal with subjects and investigations unallowed to others, yet it is with the high moral, ennobling aim of soothing or relieving humanity in its sufferings and pains, a design grand enough to submerge all passion ten times ten fathoms deep, and inspire our souls with the purest and holiest emotions. Science properly pursued is never grovelling or sensual, but soaring, elevating, religious, and the truly great or good are never demeaned thereby.

Agassiz commences his great work with a tortoise; but instead of being belittled by the seeming commonness of the theme, like a very

Atlas, he constructs a world of knowledge on that not unworthy pedestal. Science and religion elevate what else might be degrading, impart virtue to what else might be demoralizing, and in their blended lustre enable us to read touching lessons of piety and virtue, where ignorance finds occasion only for ribald jest. The physician, who prostitutes the glory of the knowledge of his profession to the nutrition of the basest passions, must of all others rank lowest and meanest of mankind, and we are glad to believe that in action the purity of our brethren will favourably compare with that of other classes of the community. Perhaps as much cannot be said of expression and conversation, and yet these are so intimately connected with thought, and feeling, and action, that they claim our most watchful regard. Words not only come from the mind, but they have a reflex power. Though they may be casual, thoughtless, momentary, they leave their imprint on the soul. No one can habitually or frequently indulge in foolish talk and obscene anecdote without an impression being made upon the inner man; and the fountain turbid only at its mouth, will ere long have its purer waters tainted by the influence. There is no one, it seems to me, in whom indecent remark is less excusable or more disgusting than in the physician. His business is to heal and hide, rather than proclaim the foibles or maladies of nature, and he lowers himself and his calling, if instead of supporting its dignity he degrades it to the nourishment of those evil communications which never fail to corrupt good manners. Low association and conversation make their mark on no one sooner than on us. They give a secret tone to character and feeling which are recognized by the chaste and sensitive; and, if we may so express it, the *pigmentum nigrum* of obscenity is often traceable in tinges and shadings imperceptible to one's self. There is something noble and exalting in the physician into whose uncontaminated heart suffering can breathe its secret accents with the history of its causes, and feel confident that medical skill combines with high minded purity in seeking to alleviate and soothe; but how different if it has reason to fear that its complaints may become the play and the sport of the next idle hour! We have been initiated into the mysteries of human life only for scientific and philanthropic purposes; and does it not become us, not only with our patients, but in each other's society, to avoid that laxity of remark with which true science and correct taste have no affinity? In the experience of the members of many medical clubs and associations, I fear there is proof of the need of reform in this last particular. It is our privilege together to enjoy the merry laugh and the proper joke; but never let us, as the manner of some is, have ever ready on our lips that jesting which is not convenient. "Let no corrupt communication proceed out of your mouth but that which is good to the use of edifying."

There are other minor temptations which might be here noticed, but we believe those already specified the chief to which our profession renders us particularly liable. The more general and manifold evil tendencies of our natures, which we mourn in common with all mankind, are considered with sufficient fulness in religious books addressed to every accountable being; and we shall now therefore more pleasantly turn from the shadows to the lights of our professional life.

CHAPTER III.

Religious privileges of the physician—brought in contact with all classes—opportunity of learning human wants—his ability to elevate the physical, intellectual, and moral condition of man—special duties to patients—how and when to exert religious influence over them—modes to which he may resort—responsibilities we are under.

It is with satisfaction we pass to the contemplation of the privileges which our profession furnishes, and the moral duties it requires of us. Education in itself confers power and imposes responsibilities which, as accountable beings, it behoves us most seriously to consider. Introduced into the inner sanctuary of nature's grand cathedral, the upgoings and outgoings of our souls should be those of holy aspiration and intense desire for good, finding vent and exercise in noble acts and loving deeds. The talent committed to our care is one for which at his coming the Lord will call us to account, and in the ledger of the present there is a debit as well as a credit side. It is a great thing to know, but greater still to apply our attainments just when and where and how they will tell most powerfully on the present and future destiny of man. It is a difficulty with much abstract learning and scientific study, that they have no ready medium through which to touch and penetrate the beating heart of the great world of practical life. Cold, ascetic, problematic, the scholar sometimes seems to wander in a region of his own, and the vast common throng of the people do not feel the thrill of any grand sympathetic nerve binding them in union real and intimate. In turn the student feels the reflex power, and, wrapping his mantle of seclusion around him, seems bound in the same leather with his books. In individual life it is easy to show the supremacy of mind over matter, but it is a problem far more intricate to demonstrate how the great intellectual and moral power of the educated shall best be brought in contact with the multitude, the masses of human kind, and make learning of practical utility to the every-day life of a moving world. Medical life, more naturally than any other business, thus utilizes education, and confers on us unusual facilities for promoting true socialism. The physician is the visitor of the world's every-day homes, has to do with the social compact, the centre of all human associations, and the radical starting point of all lasting reforms; and he sees it, not in the array or concealment of expected company, but in the plain unhidden reality of life. To him, too, are most frequently unbosomed secret sorrows, and what the eye may not discover of hidden griefs.

The only way to appreciate human degradation is to see it, and true Howards are not kept in marble palaces, nor can they even originate the best theories of human elevation surrounded by tomes of book learning. We must go into the world to learn the wants of the world. We do not, I think, feel the great opportunities we as physicians enjoy for the advancement and elevation of our race. Others are philanthropists by occasion, we have a right to consider ourselves such by profession. Thrust in amidst the different conditions of society, having to do with what in our worldly distinctions are called the highest and lowest classes; we have opportunities of comparison and reflection which will generally point out to us the chief causes of human degradation, and enable us with the best prospects of success to seek a remedy. Should the physicians of any of our large cities, for instance, collate all the facts under their own personal observation, and within the sphere of their knowledge as to the physical welfare of the people, and from actual survey propose and argue the most efficient plans of reaching and abating existing evils; what a change would it make in the sanitary and moral condition of the community! We owe it as a duty to mankind to be a self-constituted board of health, and to feel that the public are entitled to the facts with which we are familiar. Hygiene has more to do with the moral elevation of humanity than we are apt to consider. Industry, cleanliness, comfort, and health are Christian virtues; they have to do with religion as well as matter; and though true worth may exist where all these are absent, such is not the rule. Even in promoting these, in the line of our business, we contribute our proportion to the purification of social existence.

In the more direct sphere of the intellectual and moral, still greater privileges are associated with our profession. How many, by an encouraging word, a listening sympathy, a suggestive counselling, may you be the means of inducing to shake off paralyzing misanthropy, and make giant efforts to succeed! How many may you lead to forsake pernicious habits and vile associations, not by stern reproof, but by a portraiture of consequences, by the kind admonition and friendly interest of the family physician! How many may you induce to listen to the preached gospel, how many children to attend the Sabbath or day-school, how many to seek something higher than their present position! Noble institutions of charity, asylums for the aged, the widow, the orphan, the blind, the dumb, the outcast, now flourishing in this and other lands, are, in no small degree, monuments to the Christian zeal of medical men; who, in the walks of their daily practice beholding the suffering necessities of particular classes, have urged or developed the means of amelioration. We have a personal interest as members of the great brotherhood of man in every family we visit, and the question readily suggests itself in respect to many of them, How can we quietly and unobtrusively do them good? He who is on the watch for imparting priceless benefits will often, in a very easy and natural way, accomplish his object.

"The greatest discovery I ever made," said Sir Humphrey Davy, "was that of Michael Faraday in a workshop;" and many a son of poverty, yet of genius and worth, we may assist to elevate. Oh! there is something higher, nobler, more glorious, in medicine, than the efficacious pill and powder; and important as these may be, a broader land is thrown open to us, and the command is to go up and possess it; and though misery and discouragements may be in our pathway, like threatening Amalekites, they will vanish before the faithful effort. Depend upon it, we are scarcely yet commencing to know what avenues of good are incidental to our calling, and it is no vain boasting to feel the advantages we enjoy over other members of the community. In their great and praiseworthy schemes for ameliorating the condition of society, mistakes are often made by others which medical knowledge or observation would correct. The Royal Humane Society has been for years attending to the recovery of the drowned; but Marshall Hall, bringing his analysis of the reflex nervous system to bear upon the subject, has proposed a far better code of laws, and shown, that efficacious as former efforts have been, they would have accomplished still more with a different management. So acquaintance with the physical will often give us an insight into causes and sources which bear upon the moral, and teach us how best to help in saving those submerged amid the still more destructive waves of misery and sin. Ours is a humanitarian art, and morality, philanthropy, and Christianity have a right to ask at our hands more than we have as yet accomplished. Contemplate the true philosophy of life, and take time to think upon the means you enjoy of doing good, and plans and opportunities will come trooping by, eloquent in their practicability and results. In our visits to the world's homes, and in our more public influence, by promoting sound learning and religious truth, we provide at once the prophylactic and specific to human degradation, and do our part in working out the problem of human civilization and salvation.

There is a speciality in respect to the moral duties of our calling that deserves a separate consideration, and that is, how far we are called upon to pay attention to the religious interests of our immediate patients. It is a solemn thing to have a sick man die under our hands, and go to judgment unprepared. There is sometimes need of ministering to the soul as well as to the body; and sickness, when not the most severe, often serves as a milestone in the pilgrimage of life to remind us whither we are journeying, and affords a propitious occasion for drawing the attention from the business of the present to that of the future, from life to death, from time to eternity.

Man's religious nature has a claim upon us, and our peculiar position in reference to those under our immediate care, at thoughtful and critical moments, should and does lead the Christian physician to inquire into his duty as an accountable being—accountable not only for himself, but for the influence he exercises or fails to exercise upon others. Even the conscientious are frequently in doubt as to the course they should now pursue. The mind and the body act and react on each other. If the one is disturbed by allusions to the future, it may seriously affect the other, and the hope of recovery is an element which we feel like husbanding. Conversation upon religious subjects may alarm the patient, and cause fearful foreboding and misapprehension. Such difficulties and objections deserve to be weighed, and are points worthy of our thought and judgment. These excuses often seem more plausible than they are in fact. There are few who on sick beds have no solemn thoughts; our silence does not keep eternity out of view; and oftener than we think it is a relief for those morally disturbed to whisper into the ear of sympathy the feelings which agitate them. It is a comfort sometimes to unburden the mind by sharing its turbulence with a friend, and words, like tears, often afford inward peace. Religion is even better to live by than to die by, and there is a mode of approach, and a frankness of expression less likely to alarm than an apparent studied reserve. It is right for the physician to exercise his judgment in critical cases, and perhaps to prohibit serious conversation; but he should be careful to know that the perils of the case require it. It sometimes happens, when we least suspect it, that the body is already suffering from mental anguish, and thus neglect in ministering to the soul complicates the physical malady. An illustration occurring under his own observation was related to me but recently by a friend. A patient was very ill, and her physicians, although discovering her fear of death, and anxiety about her spiritual condition, forbade any communication on the subject. She gradually sank, and without any hope for the body she was encouraged to seek the welfare of her soul. Her mind grasped that medicine which is found in the balm of Gilead, the mists cleared away, and the released spirit was at rest. The physical prostration was invigorated by that godliness with contentment which is great gain; and it soon became evident that mental and moral distress had for weeks been aggravating that of the body.

There are circumstances in which the physician might not safely introduce religious themes for fear of exciting misapprehension, or from not feeling freedom to do so, in which nevertheless by a suggestion to some member of the family, or by the visit of the minister, good might be accomplished. By merely acquainting the pastor or pious friends in the community with the existing sickness, without hinting any opinion as to the result, the desired object may be attained. Where recovery is out of all question, and where we hesitate not to warn the patient to arrange his temporal concerns, in such cases, though the hope of salvation be well nigh hopeless, we need not, we ought not to omit to point to the cross, to our Saviour with arms extended for deliverance, to the necessity of preparation for that life beyond the grave.

But happily our official duties are not confined to acute death-bed sickness. It is ours oftener, and more pleasurably to see the ruddy glow of returning health, and to witness the reviving of drooping energy and reanimated strength. Now no fears of doing our patient harm by an untimely word need distress us. God's lesson of the helplessness of man, and the need of reliance upon a higher power, is fresh in illustration ; diminished pain gives better opportunity for calm and reasonable thought; the cares of the world are necessarily set aside, and the physician in his more cheerful, and less anxious visits owes to his friend, himself, and his Maker some suggestions as to the claims of Christianity. Many a one, who has feared to say a word lest it should give offence, has been surprised to find how ready and feeling a response it has met from the hearer. How easy, how proper, to casually drop a serious thought, the more touching from its informality, and thus perchance say a word in season which may give rise to a train of thought ending in celestial hopes! It has been said that the convalescent person looks upon the physician as an angel, and sure it is as a rule that no other at that time, and he at no other time, is more likely to exert a beneficial influence on his charge. It is one of the most convenient seasons we have for doing good, and a passing remark, a serious conversation, a single tract, a little book, may be the means of effecting an everlasting cure which heaven itself will celebrate, and the record of which will be found in the

Lamb's book of life. "Let the [physician] know that he which converteth the sinner from the error of his way shall save a soul from death, and shall hide a multitude of sins."

There is another class of disease in which, if any difference, our moral obligations are still more serious and pressing, and yet in which we have little reason to fear ill results from well-timed, judicious, spiritual effort. Such are those in which the malady lingers in its course, in chronic form protracting its destructive work, but with no less certainty of irremediable fatal issue. These make up no small proportion of the modes of death, and allow extended time for suggestion and reflection. Here there is absent the alarm of the sudden and acute disease, and in the most potent of all these there is a disposition just the other way, to cling to hope, to call the hectic flush the blush of health, and the occasional feeling of strength the insignia of recovery. In all these maladies, again, we have no excuse for silence, while the consciousness of experience tells us we must not delay, or death will be away with his trophy. We should not then omit or postpone to surround the patient with such influences, and impart such counsels, as, with a blessing from above, shall lead to serious contemplation. But does some physician say, that it is ours to attend to the body, not to the soul, that it is better to mind one's own business? Such was the reply not long since made to one who spoke to a friend of his immortal interests; but, as he kindly demonstrated to him how much it was his concern, he induced him to follow on until he accepted the great salvation. They who ask, Am I my brother's keeper? are often the very ones most accountable for their condition; and to us, with a patient as the subject, and approaching death as the monitor, the chiming voices of revelation and sense, of time and eternity, answer, Yes. My professional brother, let not such an one go down to the grave without your having at least asked yourself, and answered the question, whether you ought not, by conversation, by conduct, the lent book, or persuasive sympathy, to strive to lead the thoughts on high. Says the excellent Baxter, "Physicians that are much about dying men should, in a special manner, make conscience of this duty. It is their peculiar advantage that they are at hand—that they are with men in sickness and danger, when the ear is more open and the heart less stubborn than in time of health; and that men look upon their physician as a person in whose hand is their life, or, at least, who may do much to save them; and therefore they will the more regard his advice. You that are of this honourable profession, do not think this a work beside your calling, as if it belonged to none but ministers; except you think it beside your calling to be compassionate, or to be Christians. Oh help therefore, to fit your patients for heaven; and whether you see they are for life or death, teach them both how to live and die, and point them to a remedy for their souls as you do for their bodies." Even where no good results to the immediate person concerned, upon ourselves the effort brings its own reward. It reaches the ear of Him in whose hand is the book of remembrance, and it moves and refreshes the fountains of our own hearts. And when it is our privilege to converse with those upon whose souls light has dawned amid the darkness, or with others who are calmly resting on long cherished hopes; how is the valley of Baca made to us a well from which we draw spiritual draughts to fit us anew for our Christian journeying! How often too may we assist in making a religious impression, powerful and lasting, upon inmates of the same family or cherished friends! The sickness or death of those near and dear has frequently been the occasion of leading the survivors to seek for more lasting trust, and words now uttered are still more likely to foster the impression.

Afflictions are sometimes "celestial benedictions," blessings in disguise, especially if, by reading or remark, the thought be directed to that source of everlasting peace whose placid waters not a single wave of adversity shall ever ripple. Oh! it becomes us to watch for souls as those who must give an account of their stewardship, and if we rely as much upon prayer for blessing on our efforts as upon the efforts themselves, we shall not be disappointed. New elements of power for good will be developed, habit will simplify what seems difficult, and desire, tact, and experience, prevent obtrusiveness on the one hand, and neglect on the other. Let us not then be recreant to our lofty trusts, or to the noble opportunities we enjoy of assisting, under God, in delivering our fellow-men from the thraldom of ignorance and sin, and securing that eternal emancipation of the soul which owns no other kingship but the one Supreme, and no other chain but that welcome one of love, imperishable, infinite, divine.

CHAPTER IV.

Examples worthy of our imitation both in sacred and profane history—Christ the Saviour and Luke the evangelist in their earthly relations to the sick and afflicted—the practicability of combining high religious principle and professional skill and success—religious biography of Boerhaave, Hey, Good, Hope, and others as models for us.

It has been said that history is philosophy teaching by example. The remark applies with equal force to biography, and when we view the records of Christian men, the proverb is still more important and applicable. Religious experience has to do in part with the unseen and eternal. Its eye of faith penetrates a veil about which others cannot so fully reason, and the earnest, heartfelt exposition of what others have felt and known is of no little value in directing us. The testimony derived from the inward consciousness and practical life of the Christian is the best proof of the faith and principles he professes, and we may with propriety turn to the illustration and enforcement which examples afford. The religious biography of medicine is not as familiar to our profession as it should be. Divinity has its Doddridges, and Martyns, and a great host of holy exemplars; Law, its Hales and Ellsworths; the Camp, its Gardiners and Havelocks; and in our calling we are not without some guides to direct us by example as well as by precept in the way to heaven, and to exhibit to our senses how it is possible for the physician to be good as well as great. It may not be unprofitable for us to notice the religious history of a few, that we may be led to that admiration of which the highest expression is imitation. Even in the records of sacred writ, we find ourselves within the pale of medical sympathy. Among the most devoted and faithful followers of the truth as it is in Jesus, was Luke the beloved physician.

He is represented even in profane history

as a noble model of an educated Christian physician, a supposed graduate of a then noted school of medical science, in practice combining his religion with his every-day duties in beautiful and attractive symmetry. The accuracy and minuteness of his descriptions and details show that he was entirely familiar with the great events connected with Christ's advent and life; his doings and sayings; his mission and death. As he had ever with him the lineaments of his divine Master, and the cherished memory of his practice and precepts, so should we ever carry with us this pattern, and strive to be like Him that we may at last see him as he is. As Luke was a companion and ever constant friend of Paul, that model of Christian ministers, so the physician of the present day should be the supporter and aid of God's faithful messengers, encouraging them by sympathy, effort, and co-operation, instead of, as has too often been the case, making them the aim of critical remark, and open opposition.

The Gospel of Luke, and the Acts of the

apostles of which he was also the recorder, have sometimes seemed to me like the first good tidings, announced by the first Christian physician, to his profession and the world. In style admitted to be the most finished and attractive of the evangelists, with the marks of a chaste and educated mind directed by the pen of inspiration, his narratives and illustrations would, were all the rest of the Bible lost, introduce us to a complete system of religious belief and worship; and the mark of a discerning medical witness is not unfrequently manifest. He alone refers minutely to the birth of John the Baptist, and to the circumstances attending that of the babe of Bethlehem; to the miraculous cure of the woman bowed eighteen years with infirmity; to the cleansing of the ten lepers, the raising to life of the son of the widow of Nain, and to the miracles wrought by Paul. In the description of other cures referred to by other evangelists he is more specific; and the entire particulars of the death and resurrection of Christ are related by him with more extended minuteness than anywhere else. Births, diseases, cures, and deaths, form no small part of his narrative, and who better fitted than he to speak and judge of these? Thus, added to inspired authority, we have the testimony of a discriminating medical man, as if God had chosen him as a perfect and convincing medium through which to declare the history and miracles which are the abundant attestation of our holy religion. Thus a part of the divine message is conveyed to us by a competent witness from our own number, and oh that we may receive the inspired and gracious words of eternal life which he has made known unto us!

The medical man cannot, indeed, read any part of the scripture history of Christ on earth, without his thoughts being turned to contemplate him as the great Physician. By this title he refers to himself. As should we, he went about doing good; his fondest moments were often spent in the relief of suffering and want; to cure the sick, raise the dead, give sight to the blind, and bid the lame leap for joy, were the tokens of his human sympathy, and more than human power; and though clothed with that heavenly skill which forbids us to speak of him as a mere earthly healer, yet the terms applied to him as the restorer of diseased bodies, and the everlasting relief of sin-sick and burdened souls, cannot but make deep impression upon the careful medical reader; and not unfrequently do we find modes of expression, and trains of thought and action suited especially to address themselves to us. From the sacred record let us take Christ the Saviour as our heavenly, and Luke, the beloved physician, as our earthly model, and strive to walk in their most holy footsteps.

As we turn from sacred to secular biography, we are not left to trace the paths of medical life without human exemplars, in the practical exercise of their profession illustrating the symmetrical union of sound religious faith and fruitful Christian experience with high professional ability and success.

Referring back to a period long since past, foremost among those worthy of our remembrance, we find the name of the distinguished Boerhaave. With a discerning intellect, his quick perception singled out the choicest avenues of knowledge, and in the science and practice of the medical art, the fine powers of his mind found scope for healthy and vivacious expansion. Rapidly did he travel onward and upward in the royal road of fame. Successive multitudes sought relief at his hands, princes waited for his audience, and even Peter the Great is said to have tarried hours for an interview. One after another, the professorships of the University called for his services, until he arrived at the highest post of its honour. Students of Botany, Chemistry, and Medicine hastened to his presence; wealth and fame poured out their treasures before him; and as a scholar, a scientific man, and a physician, he stood aloft the wonder of his age.

But let not his medical and literary standing obscure the religious character which adorned it. Born at Leyden, in 1668, both his country and his times were such as put to the test the moral principles of men; but amid all his acquirements and reputation he sought and exemplified that "wisdom which maketh wise."

The Bible was his book of daily meditation, and to it he attributed that power of control which enabled him to preserve an equable temper amid great provocation; which made him childlike and humble amid his highest honours; and which led him to dispense with a liberal hand to the wants of the less favoured of his race. It and prayer were the sources from which he derived mental and moral vigour for the toils of his calling, and in daily life he seems to have recognized the need of divine guidance and aid. Subject at various periods to extreme suffering from imperfect respiration, cheerfulness and submission graced his social intercourse, and he practised the maxim by which as he said, living or dying, he wished to abide: "That is only best which is perfectly agreeable to the divine goodness and majesty." "God be praised," was his triumphant utterance over the pangs of disease, and having nearly reached his three score years and ten, he readily exchanged the honours of this life for the immortal crown and the eternal residence.

Ah! where the incongruity of high intellectual power and practical Christianity! What in a human existence more sublime than the mind of intelligent manhood made radiant with the light of heaven, a halo of glory encircling the massive brow, and the business, the duties, the hopes, the entire life, of the physician sanctified by the reflected effulgence of that truth whose origination and culminating point is God!

Near the close of the earthly career of Herman Boerhaave was born, on British soil, another distinguished practitioner of the healing art, to whose noble character united with the highest medical attainment, the surgeon and the Christian may pleasurably refer. William Hey early gave promise both of that intellectual and moral power, which were so forcibly and successfully developed, during the period of a life reaching to the age of eighty three.

He early became impressed with the truths of revelation, and the necessity of a personal acceptance of the plan of salvation opened up in the gospel, and after careful examination embraced it as the only guaranty of present and everlasting bliss. While pursuing his medical studies in London, we find him lamenting that he could not meet with any religious student in the same pursuit; but by his industry and correct conduct gaining an influence over those whom the same principles did not restrain. He resolved "to spare no pains to qualify himself for that state to which the providence of God had called him, and then trust him with the success of his endeavours." His experience both in his profession and in his varied relations was made up of such checkered scenes, as called into exercise all the traits of his religious nature. For long years he struggled on before his practice provided him an adequate support, until success crowned his efforts, and he became acknowledged one of the ablest surgeons of his day.

As senior surgeon of the Leeds hospital, as an honorary member of the Royal Society, and as the chief magistrate of his native city, he received his share of worldly consideration, and yet, in the faithful discharge of his duties, encountered such opposition and reproach as put to the test both his principles and faith. But severer trials marked his personal and social history. At the age of thirty-seven he received an injury which for some time incapacitated him for exertion, and, a few years after, a fall upon the thigh which threatened entirely to lay him aside from his chosen occupation, and which left him ever after seriously crippled. During the sickness to which he was subjected, and the interference which they caused to his professional labours, no words of repining or complaint issued from his lips. "If it be," said he, "the will of God that I should be confined to a sofa, and he command me to pick straws for the rest of my life, I hope I should feel no repugnance to his good pleasure."

In his family circle still more afflictive dispensations befell him. Four of his children were taken from him in early youth, and five others in succession soon after their entrance upon labours of usefulness and promising success. If any thing would seem pre-eminently capable of arousing the rebellion of nature, it is the oft repeated strokes of affliction; but the religion of this mourning father was equal to the test. On the bended knee we find him pouring out his emotions before God, blessing him that he had good reason to believe that the nine had but departed to a better world, and making his sore bereavements the occasion of rousing himself to greater zeal and devotion in the service of his Master.

Few men have ever lived, who so habitually exemplified the peace and happiness which the gospel is able to impart. With the experience of a long life, "Oh," said he, "there is no support, no comfort, but in a reliance on the atonement and intercession of the Lord Jesus Christ. Oh what a blessed thing it is to be looking unto Jesus, and resting upon the promises of God in him! 'Behold what manner of love the Father hath bestowed upon us that we should be called the sons of God.' 'If any man sin, we have an advocate with the Father, Jesus Christ the righteous; and he is the propitiation for our sins, and not for ours only, but for the sins of the whole world.'"

Such were some of his fondest quotations and contemplations; and who that does not desire such sublime reliance? Where the physician, who, with the skill and success of William Hey, would not love to add the sparkling glory of his piety? He not only, if we may so speak, died Christianity, but he lived it.

His very presence and intercourse made his patients feel that he was anxious for their spiritual as well as their temporal restoration; and his influence, though dispersed like the dew in a thousand minute and humble drops, reflected the rays of the Sun of righteousness on many a languishing soul. He departed, as he had lived, with faith, and peace, and praise, and glory, furnished by the preparation of the past; but by the night of death brought out more vividly, as the morning stars which ushered in his immortal day.

With his example brought pointedly home to us as that of an eminent brother practitioner, who will not utter the prayer, "Let me live the life of the righteous, and let me die with a refuge and a hope like his?"

Another distinguished example which may properly be commended to the physician of the present day is that of John Mason Good. It is recorded of him by his biographer that "amid all the occupations of his professional life, and all his application to literary pursuits, as a student and author, he still found time and inclination to investigate the claims of Christianity; and having become convinced of its truth and importance, he practised upon its precepts, was eventually led to embrace its doctrines, and its spirit as the great ultimatum of human attainments, and seeking for intelligence at the fountain of intellect, to find Him whom to know is life eternal." His experience is especially instructive to the sceptical. His "Book of Nature," so varied in its scope and illustration, exhibits his fondness for the wonders of earth, and from his intense enthusiasm in the search, he was temptingly exposed to the deluding charms of materialistic belief. In his primal efforts, we accordingly find him a materialist in respect to man's origin, and a universalist as to his destiny, amusing himself with finely wrought theories of creation and happiness; but the careful and candid examination of fifteen years enabled him, above and beyond, to see a light beaming through the tinted cloud which had so long beguiled his vision.

In 1815, at the meridian age of life, with his accumulated knowledge, and research into the anatomy and phenomena of animate and inanimate existence, he declared that "there was no intermediate ground upon which a sound reasoner could make a firm stand, between pure deism and modern orthodoxy as held by evangelical churches," and with zeal he embraced the latter.

O word! O wisdom! boundless theme
 Of rapture and of grief;
Lord, I believe thy truth supreme;
 Oh help my unbelief.

Such was the poetic utterance of his unreserved submission to the power of truth, and in the intense duties of his active profession, and the varied literary labours which devolved upon him, he exhibited the purity of a Christian life, and the propriety of a godly conversation. The private duties of his holy religion were not neglected, and in the following daily prayer he has left a form of petition worthy of the notice of us all. "O thou great Bestower of health, strength, and comfort! grant thy blessing upon the professional duties in which this day I may engage. Give me judgment to discern disease, and skill to treat it; and crown with thy favour the means that may be devised for recovery; for with thine assistance, the humblest instrument may succeed, as, without it, the ablest must prove unavailing. Save me from all sordid motives; and endow me with a spirit of pity and liberality towards the poor, and of tenderness and sympathy towards all; that I may enter into the various feelings by which they are respectively tried; may weep with those that weep, and rejoice with those that rejoice. And sanctify thou their souls, as well as heal their bodies. Let faith, and patience, and every Christian virtue they are called upon to exercise, have their perfect work; so that in the gracious dealings of thy Spirit and of thy providence, they may find in the end, whatever that end may be, that it has been good for them that they have been afflicted. Grant this, O heavenly Father, for the love of that adorable Redeemer, who, while on earth, went about doing good, and now ever liveth to make intercession for us in heaven. Amen."

As he drew nigh the borders of the grave, humility and faith were the befitting emblems of his greatness in the past, and his hopes for the future. "I have taken," said he, "what unfortunately the generality of Christians too much take—the middle walk of Christianity.

I have endeavoured to live up to its duties and doctrines; but I have lived below its privileges. I have been led astray by the vanity of human learning, and by the love of human applause."

His last expressions were those of trusting and overflowing love to that Saviour, whose religion had adorned his declining years; and his memory is to us a symmetrical monument of consistent piety, great ability, and high professional success. Learn from him, how these characteristics, like brethren, may dwell together in unity.

Passing on to a still more recent period, the Christian and medical standing of the distinguished stethoscopist, James Hope, commends itself to our notice. The peculiar characteristics of his mind were such, as give additional importance to his belief, with those who are not affected by the expressions of intense and excited feeling, so much as by the calm conclusions of thinking, plodding, reasoning men.

"It was a remarkable circumstance," says

one of his biographers, "in the moral history of Dr. Hope, that it was very much through the instrumentality of his reasoning powers that his heart became affected by religious subjects. He was slow in forming a conclusion on any subject, nor was ever disposed to do so, till he had fathomed depths, and probably unravelled many intricacies which to a more superficial mind would have been scarcely apparent." The same calm and deliberate investigation, which he applied to an analysis of the diseases of the heart, and to the general subject of pathological anatomy, and which enabled him to open up a new and delightful field of professional knowledge, was exercised in his examination of the claims of Christianity; and the Spirit of God blessing his search, it resulted not only in a tacit recognition, but in a decisive and unwavering acceptance of the gospel salvation.

His was the life of a devoted and consistent Christian physician; and the honours and success which attended him did not dim the bright power of his religious example. At the meridian period of life, and with a reputation constantly extending, he was attacked with those symptoms of pulmonary disease, which, while they deceive many, could in no wise mislead him. With thankfulness to God that he had not postponed his preparation to the months of sickness and decay, in a calm and steady faith he expressed his willing acquiescence in the substitution of the near prospect of heaven, for the arduous toils of his profession. "Joyfully did he resign the blessings of this world, because he found within his grasp, richer treasures, surpassing honours, purer joys, which shall never fade or cloy, but endure for ever and ever."

On the evening before his death, with an undisturbed mind, he recognized the signs of hastening dissolution. "I have," said he, "no set speeches to make, but two things to say. The first is farewell to my wife; the second is soon said, 'Christ is all and in all to me. I have no hope except in him; he is indeed all, and in all.'" Quietly, but sensibly, his powers of respiration failed; now and then some sweet passage of his blessed guide book escaping from his lips, and with thanks to God, as his last connected utterance,

> " He passed through glory's morning gate,
> And entered Paradise."

With such a model, who can feel it to be unintellectual, and unprofessional to be a Christian! Oh! does not the crown of righteousness sit gracefully and gloriously on such a brow, and does it not behove us all to choose the better part, and lay hold upon eternal life?

We have thus noticed a few of those of our own calling who, at various periods of time, and under diverse circumstances, have illustrated the noble combination of medical and moral greatness. Did space permit, it would be pleasant to portray the character of the excellent Baron Haller, with the double argument of science and revelation enforcing the reasonableness of inspired truth; Bateman, abhorring the materialism and scepticism of his early belief, and declaring that the blessing of his conversion was a "theme for his perpetual thanksgiving by day and by night;" Sir William Knighton, living religion within the walls of royalty; Parr claiming "the most desirable profession to be that of physic, because equally favourable to a man's moral sentiments and intellectual faculties;" Burder writing dutiful letters to a junior practitioner; and Bell, and Rush, and Bliss, and a host of others whose influence was on the side of truth and righteousness. More than all, there are in our own profession, in our own land, living epistles known and read of all men, whose holy lives and godly conversation furnish the vital exemplification of what the Christian physician is and ought to be. But why need we multiply examples? Those already referred to are sufficient to exhibit the practicability of combining temporal and eternal wisdom; and to present before us men of like occupation and temptations with ourselves, who are worthy models for our imitation.

Christianity, not only in theory, in reason, in nature, in revelation, commends itself to our acceptance; but human experience brings it directly home to our hearts as a practical system, and adapted to elevate intellectual talent and professional worth, and to secure that happiness which surrounds the very business of life with a sheen of satisfaction, hides the grimness of death beneath the smiles of hope, and inspires the soul with the sustaining prospect of an ever radiant immortality.

CONCLUSION.

In the preceding pages we have briefly noticed the tendency of the study and practice of medicine, the temptations to which it exposes us, the privileges it confers, and a few of the examples which exhibit its practical combination with Christianity. It has not been our aim to compass the whole field of argument and illustration; but rather to open up a fountain of thought, flowing out by natural contemplation into a thousand rivulets, conferring power, health, and elevation both upon the thinker himself, and those with whom he is associated. Be assured we stand upon a pinnacle of that everlasting temple, whose inner court is the holy of holies; and education, opportunity, and duty, like three veritable graces, with joined hands and melodious voices, bid us do something which shall contribute to the civilization, reformation, and eternal salvation of a sinful world.

Every medical reader, whom I address, has already arranged himself in one or the other of the only two classes of candidates for immortal existence; those by the Christian faith prepared for everlasting happiness, or those with dreadful alternative, without hope, and without God in the world; unmoved as they see others gliding into the tomb, and themselves at last without a gleam of light, groping on until they fall into the immeasurable abyss. Consider, I beseech you, your imperiled destiny. It will not answer, to content ourselves with earthly perfection in an art which the happy spirit will have no need of preserving in another world; and it only adds interest, and light, and science to our pleasing pursuit, if we study it in its religious bearing. With the word of God as your guide, the book of nature and your professional knowledge as your prompters, and an earnest and prayerful desire after truth, you will not fail to find the doctor's great Physician with whom is ever to be found the elixir of life.

If we have already united the profession of the Christian with the profession of medicine, on us the claims of our united professions press with a serious responsibility. Our own spiritual vigour, and the wants of a perishing world require us to gird ourselves afresh, and awake in the strength of our Redeemer. To be good, to do good, to get good, should be our motto. The measure of opportunity is the measure of duty, and let us weigh well the accountability to which our medical profession subjects us. Trace its avenues of benefit, its motives for philanthropy, its relationship to reform, its humanitarian and social elements, its moral philosophy, its religious aspects, the inherent practicability of its power for good; and devote yourself to the improvement of its loftiest and holiest privileges by expanding them into an actual practice. Thus your days will be the witness of greater achievements than intellect can boast, and crown everlasting ages with the trophies of unfading, imperishable glory.

These pages, designedly few, I commend to your thoughtful perusal and expansive application; and though they be but as the mustard seed which is the least of all the seeds, God grant that they may be blessed to the benefit of the medical reader, and be made an humble instrumentality in preparing us for toil and duty here, and for that world where sickness and pain shall never come; where physician and patient in joyful triumph together may sing, "O death, where is thy sting? O grave, where is thy victory?" "Thanks be to God which giveth us the victory through our Lord Jesus Christ." "Let us hear the conclusion of the whole matter: Fear God and keep his commandments; for this is the whole of man. For God shall bring every work into judgment, with every secret thing, whether it be good or whether it be evil."

www.ingramcontent.com/pod-product-compliance
Lightning Source LLC
LaVergne TN
LVHW021428110826
845150LV00007B/2136

9781425507299